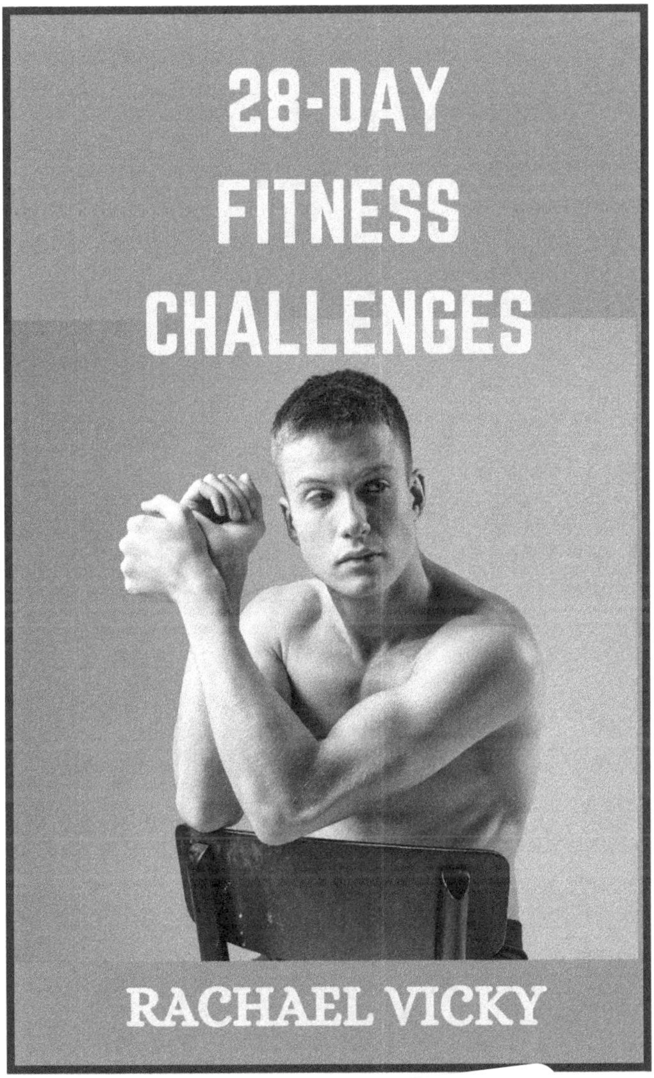

28-DAY FITNESS CHALLENGES

RACHAEL VICKY

INTRODUCTION

CHAPTER 1

SET SMART GOALS

CHAPTER 2

28-DAY TRAINING PLAN

CHAPTER 3

NUTRITION FOR FITNESS

CHAPTER 4

UPGRADE YOUR PLATE: Restaurant Tips and Tricks

CHAPTER 5

STRENGTH TRAINING FOR BEGINNERS

   Bodyweight exercises sample for beginners

CHAPTER 6

MOVING ON-week 4 of challenge

CHAPTER 7

YOU DID IT!-celebrate success and look to the future

INDEX

INTRODUCTION

Welcome to the 28 Day Fitness Challenge!

Are you ready to start your fitness journey?, feel energized and see positive changes in your body and mind?

This challenge is designed to guide you through the next four weeks, filled with effective exercises, helpful tips and the motivation you need to succeed.

What to expect after 28 days In this program, you'll embark on a progressive workout plan that challenges and improves your overall fitness.

We will focus on a variety of exercises including strength training, cardio, core work and mobility to create a comprehensive foundation for your health.

Here's what you can expect: **Structured Daily Workouts:** Each day will include a specific workout routine designed to target different muscle groups and improve your heart health.

Clear Instructions: Each exercise will come with detailed descriptions, sets, repetitions and rest periods to ensure that you perform the movements correctly and effectively.

Progression Tips: As you get stronger, we'll give you tips on how to increase the difficulty of your exercises, keeping you challenged throughout the program.

Focus on proper form: Safety first.

We will emphasize proper form for all exercises to minimize the risk of injury.

Develop Healthy Habits: This program goes beyond exercise.

We will provide information on how to eat healthy, stay hydrated and get enough rest for optimal results.

Is this challenge right for you?

This 28-day fitness challenge is designed to suit a variety of fitness levels.

Whether you are a beginner or someone looking to kick-start your fitness routine, this program can be tailored to your needs.

Here's how to know if this challenge is right for you: You're motivated to improve your overall health and fitness.

You are willing to commit to exercising almost every day of the week.

You are willing to learn new exercises and modify them if necessary.

You're excited about establishing healthy habits that last more than 28 days.

If you answered yes to these points then this challenge is the perfect way to start your fitness journey and discover the incredible benefits of exercise!

Get Started Now that you're excited to embark on this 28-day fitness challenge, get ready for success!

This section provides the necessary tools and knowledge to ensure you have a smooth and rewarding experience.

CHAPTER 1

SET SMART GOALS

The first step is to set clear goals to stay focused and motivated throughout the challenge.

Specific: Identify exactly what you want to achieve.

Instead of "getting stronger," aim to "increase your strength by doing 3 sets of 10 squats with proper form before the challenge ends.

Measurable: Track your progress!

Use data points like weight lifted, distance traveled, or improved endurance to quantify your achievements.

Achievable: Be realistic.

Set ambitious but achievable goals to avoid discouragement.

Related: Your goals should align with your overall fitness aspirations.

Do you want to build muscle, improve endurance or increase flexibility?

Time limit: Set a deadline for each goal.

Doing 3 sets of 10 squats at the end of the challenge will create a sense of urgency and accomplishment.

Prepare for success: Tips and equipment Here are some practical tips for preparing for success:

Create a workout space: Find a private space indoors or outside where you can comfortably do your exercises.

Gather equipment (or find an alternative): Depending on the exercise you've chosen, you may need light weights, resistance bands, a yoga mat, or an exercise ball.

However, most exercises can be modified using body weight or household items for beginners.

Choose appropriate clothing: Choose comfortable, breathable clothing that allows free movement.

Invest in a suitable pair of shoes to support your body during exercise.

Meal Plan (Optional) We will provide you with a sample meal plan (with options for vegetarians, vegans, etc.

) that emphasizes diet Eat a balanced diet rich in essential nutrients to fuel your workouts and promote recovery.

Remember that this is just a guide.

Feel free to adjust it to your preferences and dietary needs.

Avoid injury: Warm up, relax and rest safely first.

Here's how to prevent injury and ensure optimal recovery: **Warm-up:** Prepare your body for exercise with 5 to 10 minutes of light cardio (jogging, jumping jacks) and

Dynamic stretching (arm circles, leg swings) to increase blood flow and improve flexibility.

Cooldown: Spend 5-10 minutes doing static stretching (hold the stretch for 20-30 seconds) to cool your muscles and avoid soreness.

Rest: Schedule rest days to allow your body to recover and rebuild muscle tissue.

Aim for at least one rest day per week and listen to your body when it needs extra recovery time.

By following these tips and setting clear goals, you'll be well on your way to a successful and rewarding 28-day fitness challenge!

We'll go deeper into specific exercises in the next section: 28-Day Workout Plan!

CHAPTER 2

28-DAY TRAINING PLAN

Welcome to the roadmap for the next four weeks!

This chapter gets to the heart of the 28-Day Fitness Challenge: daily workouts.

We will guide you through a progressive program designed to build strength, improve endurance and leave you feeling energized and accomplished.

WEEK1: Building your foundation This week is all about building a strong foundation.

We will focus on mastering basic exercises that target major muscle groups and prepare the body for the challenges ahead.

Remember, proper form is important!

Pay attention to the descriptions and don't hesitate to modify the exercises if necessary.

MONDAY: Whole body strength Warm up (5 minutes): Light cardio like jumping rope or jogging to get blood circulating, followed by stretching movements (arm circles, leg rotations) to improve toughness.

Exercise program: Squats (3 sets, 10 reps, rest 30 seconds): Stand with your feet shoulder-width apart, toes slightly turned out.

Lower your body as if you were sitting in a chair, keeping your back straight and your muscles tense.

Push through your heels to return to standing.

Push-ups (modified or full push-ups, do 3 sets as many times as possible with good form, rest 30 seconds): If push-ups are difficult, start with your knees.

In a high plank position (body forms a straight line from head to heels), lower your torso to the floor, keeping your elbows close to your body.

Push back to the starting position.

Lunges (3 sets, 10 reps on each leg, rest 30 seconds): Step one foot forward, lowering your hips until both knees are bent at a 90-degree angle.

Return to the starting position and repeat with the other leg.

Plank (3 sets of 30-second holds, 30-second rest): Forearms on the floor, elbows shoulder-width apart, body forming a straight line from head to heels.

Engage your core and glutes to maintain this position.

Rows (using body weight, resistance bands or dumbbells, 3 sets of 12 reps, 30 seconds rest): Anchor yourself under the barbell or with a resistance band, keeping your back straight and muscles tight.

Bring your elbows back, squeezing your shoulder blades together.

Controlled descent.

Cool down (5 minutes): Static stretching exercises such as hamstring stretches, quadriceps stretches, and chest openers to improve flexibility and reduce muscle soreness.

TUESDAY: Cardio & Core Warm-up (5 minutes): Same as Monday.

Cardio: Aim for 30 minutes of moderate-intensity cardio.

This could be brisk walking, jogging, swimming, cycling or any activity that increases your heart rate and gets you moving.

Basic moves: Crunches (3 sets, 15 reps, 30 seconds rest): Lie on your back with your knees bent and feet flat on the floor.

Try to lift your upper back off the floor, bringing your chin toward your chest.

Controlled descent.

Russian Twists (3 sets of 12 reps, rest 30 seconds): Sit on the floor with your knees bent and feet flat.

Lean back slightly, keeping your body tense and your back straight.

Rotate your torso from side to side, bringing your hands to touch the floor while alternating sides.

Side plank (3 sets, hold 30 seconds, rest 30 seconds): Lie on your side with one elbow directly under your shoulder.

Lift hips off the floor in a straight line from head to heels.

Engage your core and hold on.

Switch sides and repeat.

Cooldown (5 minutes): Static stretching focuses on your core and the major muscle groups used during cardio.

WEDNESDAY: Rest and active recovery Today is your rest day!

This allows your body to recover and rebuild muscle tissue.

Consider an optional active recovery session like yoga, light stretching or walking to stay mentally relaxed.

THURSDAY: Lower body strength Warm up (5 minutes): Get blood flowing and relax your lower body with light cardio exercises and stretches like leg swings and hand rotations.

Workout route: Squats (3 sets of 12 reps, 30 seconds rest): Similar to Monday's format but increase the number of repetitions for a greater challenge.

Step-Ups (3 sets of 10 reps, rest 30 seconds):   Find a sturdy chair or step.

Stand on the bench with one leg, bringing the other knee toward your chest.

Down and Thursday: Lower-body strength (continued)   Step-ups (3 sets, 10 reps on each leg, 30 seconds rest): Find a sturdy bench or step.

Stand on the bench with one leg, bringing the other knee toward your chest.

Lower and repeat with the other leg.

Bulgarian Split Squats (3 sets, 10 reps/leg, rest 30 seconds): Stand with one leg behind you, resting your feet on a bench or chair.

Lower your body with your front leg bent at a 90-degree angle.

Return to the starting position and repeat with the other leg.

(Modified: perform regular lunges if necessary) Glute Bridges (3 sets of 15 reps, rest 30 seconds): Lie on your back with your knees bent and feet flat on the floor.

Lift your hips off the floor, squeezing your glutes at the top. Controlled descent.

Calf raises (3 sets, 15 reps, rest 30 seconds): Stand on your toes, lifting your heels off the floor.

Hold for a second at the top, then lower in a controlled manner.

You can do this exercise with your body weight or by holding dumbbells in your hands.

Cool down (5 minutes): Static stretching focuses on your quadriceps, hamstrings, glutes, and calves.

FRIDAY: Upper Body and Core Warm-up (5 minutes): Similar to Monday's warm-up, focus on relaxing the upper body with arm rotations and shoulder rolls.

Workout route: Push-ups (modified or full push-ups, 3 sets of as many reps as possible with good form, 30 seconds rest): Same as Monday.

Overhead Press (using body weight, dumbbells or resistance bands, 3 sets of 10 reps each set, 30 seconds rest): Stand with your feet shoulder-width apart, stretching your muscles.

Press the weights directly above your head until your arms are straight.

Controlled descent.

(Modified: Arnold Press: rotate your wrists as you press the weight overhead) Rows (using body weight, resistance bands or dumbbells, 3 sets of 12 reps, rest 30 seconds): Like Monday.

Bicep curl exercise (using dumbbells or resistance bands, 3 sets, 12 reps each set, 30 seconds rest): Stand with your feet shoulder-width apart, stretch your muscles.

Curl the weights toward your shoulders, squeezing your biceps at the top.

Controlled descent.

(Modified: perform hammer curls with palms facing in) Triceps exercise (use a chair or bench, do 3 sets as many times as possible with good form, rest 30 seconds): Sit on the edge of a chair or bench with your arms shoulder-width apart at your sides.

Lower your body by bending your elbows, keeping your back close to the chair.

Push back to the starting position.

Basic Routine: Plank (3 sets, hold 45 seconds, rest 30 seconds): Same as

Monday, but increase the hold time for added challenge.

Russian Twists (3 sets, 15 reps each side, rest 30 seconds): Same as Tuesday, but increase the number of reps per side.

Cool down (5 minutes): Static stretching focuses on chest, shoulders, triceps, biceps and core.

SATURDAY AND SUNDAY: Rest These are days of complete rest.

Let your body recover and recharge for a great start to week 2!

Consider light activity like walking or gentle stretching if you feel restless.

Remember. This is just an example structure.

Feel free to modify the exercises based on your fitness level and equipment availability.

Listen to your body and take rest days if necessary.

Congratulations on completing week 1!

By following these exercises and incorporating adequate rest, you will easily achieve your fitness goals.

Week 2 will introduce new exercises and increase intensity to continue to challenge yourself.

Keep stable!

WEEK 2: Increase Intensity This week builds on the foundation established in Week 1.

We'll introduce new exercises and increase the difficulty of existing ones to continue to challenge your body and encourage progress.

Remember, good form is still important!

MONDAY: Total Body Strength

Warm-up (5 minutes): Light cardio and dynamic stretching to prepare the body.

Workout routine: Squats (3 sets, 15 repetitions, 30 seconds rest): Same format as previous weeks, but increases the number of repetitions for added challenge.

Walking Lunges (3 sets, 12 reps on each leg, rest 30 seconds): Take a big step forward with one leg, lowering your hips until both knees are bent at a 90-degree angle.

Return to the starting position and repeat with the other leg.

Overhead Press (using dumbbells, dumbbells or resistance bands, 3 sets of 12 reps, 30 seconds rest): Same as week 1.

Renegade Rows (3 sets of 10 reps, 30 seconds rest): Start in a high plank position with your hands directly under your shoulders.

Lower one hand to the floor next to your chest, keeping your body in a straight line.

Return to plank position and repeat with the other hand.

Glute Bridges with Leg Extension (3 sets, 12 reps per leg, rest 30 seconds): Do a glute bridge (as in Week 1) but extend one leg toward the ceiling at the top of the movement.

Lower back down under control and repeat with the other leg.

Cooldown (5 minutes): Static stretching focuses on the major muscle groups used during the workout.

TUESDAY: Cardio & Core Warm-up (5 minutes): Same as Monday.

Cardio: Aim for 35 minutes of moderate-intensity cardio (brisk walking, jogging, swimming, cycling).

Basic routine: Plank with shoulder taps (3 sets of 30-second taps, 30-second rest): In plank position, tap one hand on opposite shoulder, then return Back to the table.

Alternate sides in a controlled manner.

Russian Twists with Medicine Ball (3 sets, 15 reps on each side, 30 seconds rest): Same as Russian Twists in Week 1, but hold a medicine ball (or weight) for added challenge.

Bird-Dogs (3 sets of 10 reps, rest 30 seconds): Start on all fours with hands shoulder-width apart and knees hip-width apart.

Extend one arm and the opposite leg, keeping your back straight and your core tense.

Lower back to the starting position and repeat on the other side.

Cooldown (5 minutes): Static stretching focuses on your core and the major muscle groups used during cardio.

WEDNESDAY: Active rest and recovery Have a nice day of rest! Consider yoga, gentle stretching, or walking to relax.

THURSDAY: Lower body and core strength Warm up (5 minutes): Focus on warming up your lower body with light cardio exercises and stretches like leg swings and lunges with a bracelet.

Workout Routine: Jump Squats (3 sets of 10 reps, 30 seconds rest): Perform a regular squat, then explode upward into a short jump at the top.

Land softly and immediately lower yourself into a squat position for the next repetition.

Bulgarian Dumbbell Split Squats (3 sets, 12 reps on each leg, 30 seconds rest): Same as Week 1, but with a dumbbell in each hand.

Hamstring Curls (3 sets, 15 reps, 30 seconds rest): Lie on your back with your knees bent and feet flat on the floor.

Lift your hips off the floor, squeezing your hamstrings to bring your heels toward your buttocks. Controlled descent.

(Modified: perform this exercise on an exercise ball for added difficulty) Step Calf Raises (3 sets, 15 repetitions per leg, 30-second rest): Stand on a step with toes over the edge.

Lower your heels to the bottom of the step, then stand on your tiptoes.

You can do this exercise with your body weight or by holding dumbbells in your hands.

Climbing (3 sets of 30 seconds, rest 30 seconds): Start in a high plank position.

Bring one knee toward your chest in a running motion, then quickly switch legs.

Maintain a good basic level of engagement throughout.

FRIDAY: Upper body strength Warm-up (5 minutes): Similar to Monday's warm-up, focus on relaxing the upper body with arm rotations and shoulder rolls.

Workout route: Push-ups (modified push-ups or full push-ups, 3 sets as many times as possible with good form, 30 seconds rest): Same as previous weeks.

Dumbbell Rows (3 sets of 12 reps, rest 30 seconds): Stand with your feet shoulder-width apart, tense your core and hold a dumbbell in each hand.

Pull the dumbbells to your sides, squeezing your shoulder blades together.

Controlled descent.

Dips (using parallel bars or a sturdy bench, 3 sets of as many reps as possible with good form, rest 30 seconds): Perform dips on a parallel bar or sturdy bench, lowering body by bending the elbows and keeping the back close to the support.

Push back to the starting position.

(Modified: perform triceps curls using a chair as in week 1) Bicep curls (3 sets, 12 reps per arm, 30 seconds rest): Stand with feet shoulder-width apart, One hand placed on a stable surface on the floor for support.

Use your other hand to curl the weight toward your shoulder, focusing on squeezing your biceps at the top.

Lower under control and repeat with the other arm.

Lateral Raises (3 sets, 15 reps each, 30 seconds rest): Stand with feet shoulder-width apart, stretch and hold dumbbells in each hand.

Raise your arms out to the sides until they are parallel to the floor, keeping your elbows slightly bent.

Controlled descent.

Cool down (5 minutes): Static stretching focuses on chest, shoulders, triceps, biceps and core.

Saturday & Sunday: Rest Take advantage of these days of complete rest to let your body recover and recharge for week 3!

Consider light activity like walking or gentle stretching if you feel restless.

This is the end of week 2 of the training program.

By following this structure, we can effectively map out the remaining workouts in weeks 3 and 4, maintaining a clear and consistent schedule throughout the 28 days.

CHAPTER 3

NUTRITION FOR FITNESS

Fueling your fitness journey goes beyond hitting the gym.

Good nutrition plays a vital role in optimizing your training, recovery and achieving your fitness goals.

This chapter covers the fundamentals of building a healthy diet and staying hydrated, and provides a sample meal plan to help you get started.

Building a healthy plate Imagine your plate divided into sections.

To create balanced meals, try adding the following key nutrients to these portions: Carbohydrates (40-50% of your diet): Carbohydrates provide the body with energy Friend.

Choose complex carbohydrates found in whole grains (brown rice, quinoa, whole grain bread), fruits and vegetables.

They provide sustained energy and fiber needed for digestion.

Limit simple carbohydrates such as sugary drinks and refined grains (white bread, pastries).

Protein (20-30% of your diet): Protein is essential for building and repairing muscle tissue.

Aim for lean sources of protein such as grilled chicken or fish, legumes (beans, lentils) and tofu (for vegetarians/vegetarians).

Healthy fats (20-30% of your diet): Don't be afraid of fat!

Healthy fats are essential for hormone regulation, cell function, and feelings of fullness.

Include healthy fats from sources such as avocados, nuts, olive oil, and oily fish (salmon, tuna).

Micronutrients Material While macronutrients (carbohydrates, proteins, fats) provide energy, micronutrients (vitamins and minerals) play an essential role in body differences.

Try to eat a variety of fruits, vegetables, and whole grains to ensure you're getting a variety of vitamins and minerals.

A Visual Guide To A Healthy Meal

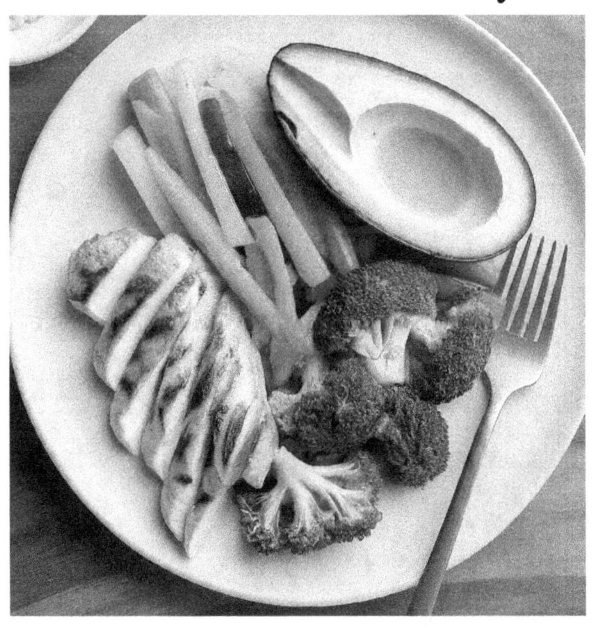

Hydration: Your body's best friend Water is essential for every function of the body, including temperature regulation, nutrient transport nourishes and lubricates joints.

Dehydration can negatively impact your exercise performance and recovery.

Here is a general guide to daily water intake: Moderate activity level: Aim to drink 2 to 3 liters (8 to 12 cups) of water each day.

High activity level: Aim to drink 3 to 4 liters (12 to 16 cups) of water each day.

Remember that these are only recommendations.

Adjust your water intake based on factors such as climate, activity level and personal needs.

If your urine is dark yellow, it's a sign you need to drink more water.

Sample meal plan (many variations available) This sample meal plan provides guidance on balanced meals throughout the day.

Feel free to adjust serving sizes and ingredients based on your calorie needs and preferences.

Breakfast (7: 00 hours): **Choice 1:** Scrambled eggs with spinach and whole grain toast, berries on the side.

Choice 2: Greek yogurt with berries, granola and honey.

Option 3 (vegetarian): Oatmeal with nuts, seeds and a little plant milk.

Lunch (1: 00 PM): **Choice 1:** Grilled chicken breast sandwich on whole grain bread with lettuce, tomato and avocado.

Choice 2: Salmon with grilled vegetables (broccoli, asparagus) and brown rice.

Option 3 (vegan): Lentil soup with salad and whole-wheat crackers.

Snack (15: 00 PM): A handful of almonds and dried fruit.

Apples with a spoonful of peanut butter.

Cheese with chopped vegetables.

Dinner (7: 00 PM): **Choice 1:** Stir-fried grilled tofu with vegetables and brown rice.

Choice 2: Turkey Chili and Side Salad.

Choice 3 (Vegetarian): Black bean sandwich on whole grain bread with sweet potato fries.

Snack (before bed, optional): Small cup of Greek yogurt with berries.

A handful of mixed nuts.

Variations: Vegetarian: Replace meat with tofu, tempeh, lentils or beans for a source of protein.

Vegan: Choose plant-based milks, tofu and exclude honey.

Make sure you get enough vitamin B12 through fortified foods or supplements.

Gluten-free: Choose gluten-free alternatives to breads, crackers, and pasta.

Remember: This is just a sample plan.

Feel free to explore different healthy recipes and customize the plan to your liking.

CHAPTER 4

UPGRADE YOUR PLATE:
Restaurant Tips and Tricks

Building a healthy foundation with balanced meals is important, but sometimes you crave variety or find yourself dining out.

This chapter provides inspirational recipes and restaurant survival tips to keep you on track.

Recipe inspiration: Quick and easy meal Lemon garlic chicken with pan-roasted vegetables (serves 4): **Ingredients:** 4 boneless, skinless chicken breasts 1 head broccoli, cut into florets 1 pint cherry tomatoes 1 red onion cut into florets 1/4 cup olive oil 2 tablespoons lemon juice 2 cloves garlic, chopped 1 teaspoon oregano dry 1/2 teaspoon salt 1/4 teaspoon black pepper

Instructions: Preheat oven to 400°F (200°C).

In a large bowl, mix chicken breasts with olive oil, lemon juice, garlic, oregano, salt and pepper.

Add broccoli, cherry tomatoes and cubed red onion to the bowl and drizzle with dressing.

Spread chicken and vegetables on a baking tray in a single layer.

Bake for 20 to 25 minutes or until chicken is cooked through and vegetables are tender.

Creamy pasta with tomatoes, spinach and sundried tomatoes (serves 4):

Ingredients: 1 tablespoon olive oil 1 onion, chopped 2 cloves garlic, chopped 1 can (28 ounces) diced tomatoes, undrained 1 cup vegetable broth 1/2 cup heavy cream (or herbal substitute) 1 tablespoon dried Italian herbs Salt and pepper to taste 12 ounces whole grain pasta 4 cups baby spinach 1/2 cup chopped sun-dried tomatoes (optional) Grated Parmesan cheese, to serve (optional)

Instructions: Cook the pasta Follow the instructions on the 'packaging'.

Meanwhile, heat the olive oil in a large skillet over medium heat.

Add onion and cook until soft, about 5 minutes.

Stir in the garlic and cook for another minute.

Add diced tomatoes, vegetable broth and Italian herbs.

Bring to a boil and cook for 10 minutes.

Stir in heavy cream (or plant-based alternative) and season to taste with salt and pepper.

Once the noodles are cooked, drain and add to the sauce along with the spinach and sundried tomatoes (if using).

Stirred.

Serve with grated parmesan (optional).

Spiced Green Bean Buddha Bowl (serves 2):

Ingredients: 1 can (15 ounces) green beans, drained and rinsed 1 tablespoon olive oil 1 teaspoon flour curry 1/2 teaspoon cumin 1/4 teaspoon paprika Salt and pepper to taste 2 cups cooked brown rice or quinoa 1 cucumber, chopped 1 red pepper, chopped small 1 pint cherry tomatoes, halved 1/4 cup crumbled feta cheese (optional) Tahini sauce, for drizzling .

Instructions: Preheat oven to 400°F (200°C).

Mix green beans with olive oil, curry powder, cumin, paprika, salt and pepper.

Spread the green beans on a baking tray in a single layer.

Bake for 20 minutes or until golden and crispy.

While the green beans roast, prepare your bowl by adding cooked brown rice or quinoa to the bottom.

Garnish with chopped cucumbers, bell peppers, cherry tomatoes and roasted green beans.

Drizzle with tahini and sprinkle with crumbled feta cheese (optional).

Conquer restaurant menus: Eat healthy at restaurants Eating out doesn't have to sabotage your health goals.

Here's your guide to making smart choices: Know the menu: Check menus online in advance.

Look for options with grilled or grilled proteins, whole grains, and lots of vegetables.

Changemaster: Don't be afraid to ask!

Ask for extra sauces and dressings on the side, choose whole grain bread or brown rice instead of white, and ask about portion sizes.

Serving patrol: Share a meal with friends or take half home if you have leftovers.

Beware of hidden dangers: Watch out for hidden sugars and unhealthy fats.

Sauces, salad dressings, and fried foods may contain more calories.

Ask about ingredients and preparation methods if in doubt.

Drink Smart: Avoid sugary drinks like soda and juice.

Choose water, unsweetened iced tea or black coffee.

Remember: Consistency is key.

By making wise choices and incorporating healthy habits, you can confidently navigate restaurant menus and maintain your fitness goals.

CHAPTER 5

STRENGTH TRAINING FOR BEGINNERS

Building strength is the foundation of any fitness journey.

This chapter delves into the world of strength training, guiding you through the essential bodyweight exercises and proper form to establish a solid foundation for your workout.

Why is strength training important?

Strength training offers many benefits beyond building muscle.

Here are some key reasons to incorporate it into your routine:

Boosts metabolism: Muscles burn

more calories at rest, helping with weight control and overall fitness.

Improve bone density: Strength training helps prevent bone loss and reduces the risk of osteoporosis.

Improve Daily Activities: Daily tasks become easier as strength increases, from carrying groceries to climbing stairs.

Core Strengthening: A strong core helps improve posture, stability and reduce back pain.

Build confidence: Seeing your body become stronger and more capable can be incredibly empowering.

Get started with bodyweight exercises Bodyweight exercises require no equipment and can be done anywhere, making them perfect for beginners.

Here are some basic exercises that target the major muscle groups:

Squats: A classic exercise to strengthen your legs and core.

Stand with your feet shoulder-width apart, toes pointing slightly outward.

Lower your body as if you were sitting in a chair, keeping your back straight and your muscles tense.

Push back to the starting position.

Lungs: Great for working your legs and glutes.

Step one foot forward, lowering your hips until both knees are bent at a 90-degree angle.

Return to the starting position and repeat with the other leg.

Pumps: Modify them if necessary!

Start kneeling, arms shoulder-width apart, body forming a straight line from head to heels.

Lower your chest toward the floor, then raise it to the starting position.

Row: Target your back muscles.

Find a sturdy surface like a table or bench.

Place your hands shoulder-width apart and lower your body in a straight line, keeping your body active.

Return to the starting position.

Board: Great for core strength.

Get into a high plank position with your forearms on the floor and your body forming a straight line.

Hold for as long as possible with good posture.

Master Proper Form Proper form is critical to maximizing the benefits of strength training and preventing injury.

Here are some general tips: Focus on quality over quantity: It's better to do fewer repetitions with correct form than more repetitions with incorrect form.

Maintain a neutral spine: Keep your back straight and focused throughout the exercise.

Breathe properly: Forcefully exhale and inhale as you return to the starting position.

No bouncing or jerking: Use controlled movements for a safer, more effective workout.

Listen to your body: If you feel pain, stop exercising and consult a healthcare professional if necessary.

Building a Workout Routine for Beginners Below is an example of a workout routine that combines the exercises mentioned above.

Perform 2 to 3 sets of 10 to 15 repetitions for each exercise, resting 30 to 60 seconds between sets and exercises.

Remember, this is just a starting point.

Gradually increase difficulty as you get stronger.

Bodyweight exercises sample for beginners

Monday and Wednesday: Focus on the lower body Squats (3 sets of 10 to 15 repetitions) Lunges (3 sets of 10 to 15 repetitions each leg) Glute Bridges (3 sets , 10 to 15 repetitions) Advanced hip raises (3 sets, 15-20 repetitions)

Tuesday and Thursday: Focus on the upper body Push-ups (modified push-ups or push-ups full, 3 sets of as many reps as possible with good form) Row (3 sets of 10-15 repetitions) Plank (3 sets of holds for 30-60 seconds) Warm-up and relaxation Remember!

Warm-up (5 minutes): Do light cardio like jumping rope or jogging, followed by dynamic stretches to prepare your muscles for movement.

Cooldown (5 minutes): Static stretching to improve flexibility and reduce post-workout soreness.

Embrace the journey!

Strength training is a journey, not a destination.

Be patient, consistent, and celebrate your progress.

As you get stronger, explore variations of these exercises or consider adding light weights for added challenge.

With dedication, you will build a solid foundation to be healthier and more confident.

CHAPTER 6

MOVING ON-*week 4 of challenge*

Welcome to Week 4! By now, you have established a solid exercise routine and your body is adapting to the demands of the program. This week we'll increase the intensity and challenge you with new exercises to keep pushing your limits and maximize your progress.

Remember: Good fitness is still important throughout your workout.

Feel free to adjust the weight or modify the exercises if necessary.

Sample Workout Routine (Week 4): This sample routine provides a structure you can follow during Week 4.

Remember to perform a proper warm-up (5 minutes) with light, dynamic cardio exercises before each workout session and cool down (5 minutes) with static stretching exercises afterward.

Monday: Strength & Core Squats (3 sets, 18 reps, 30 seconds rest): You can add light weights (dumbbells or kettlebells) to increase the challenge.

Walking lunges with overhead presses (3 sets of 15 reps per leg on press, rest 30 seconds): Combine lunges with overhead presses using dumbbells or dumbbells for a full-body challenge.

Bulgarian Split Squats (3 sets, 12 reps per leg, 30 seconds rest): This squat variation targets each leg individually, improving balance and stability.

Push-ups (modified push-ups or full push-ups, do 3 sets as many times as possible with good form): If full push-ups are difficult, do them on your knees.

Plank leg lifts (3 sets, 30 seconds each set, alternating between leg raises, 30 seconds rest): Maintain plank position and lift one leg off the floor one at a time.

Russian Twists with Medicine Ball (optional heavy weight) (3 sets of 18 reps, 30 seconds rest): Increase reps in Week 2 for more core challenge.

Tuesday: Cardiovascular & Flexibility Cardio: Aim for 40 minutes of moderate-intensity cardio (brisk walking, jogging, swimming, cycling).

Flexibility routine (hold each stretch for 10 - 15 minutes): Hamstring stretch: Sit on the floor with your legs straight and reach for your toes.

Quad Stretch: Stand on one leg and pull the other leg toward your butt.

Calf Stretch: Lean against the wall with your arms shoulder-width apart and one leg stretched behind you with your foot flexed.

Press your heels into the wall to feel a stretch in your calves.

Chest Stretch: Stand in front of the door and place your forearms on either side of the frame.

Lean forward to feel the stretch in your chest.

Shoulder Stretch: Clasp your hands behind your back and gently raise your arms above your head.

Wednesday: Active rest and recovery Have a nice day of rest!

Consider activities like yoga, light stretching, or walking to stay relaxed and promote recovery.

Thursday: Total body strength Deadlifts (using body weight, dumbbells or kettlebells, 3 sets of 12 reps, 30 seconds rest): Stand with feet hip-width apart, rotate body at your hips to lower the weights to the floor, keeping your back straight and engaged.

Walking lunges with bicep curls (3 sets of 15 reps per leg with curls, rest 30 seconds): Combine lunges with bicep curls by using weights to interact with the upper body.

Side Plank (3 sets, hold 30 seconds each, rest 30 seconds): Stand on one elbow in a side plank position, hips stacked and core stretched.

Renegade Rows with Dumbbell Rows (3 sets, 12 reps per side for rebel rows, 12 reps per arm for dumbbell rows, rest 30 seconds): Alternate between renegade rows and dumbbell rows to Stimulate back workout.

Single-leg glute bridge (3 sets of 15 reps on each leg with pulse, rest 30 seconds): Perform the glute bridge as before, but at the top of the movement, lift one heel off the ground and push it up.

and returned several times before returning.

Repeat with the other leg.

Friday: Cardio HIIT Workout (20 minutes): Alternate between high-intensity activity periods (sprints, jumping jacks, crunches) and low-intensity recovery periods (walking, jogging).

Aim for 30 seconds of intense exercise, then 30 seconds of rest.

Repeat this cycle for 10 minutes.

Remember: This is just an example of a habit.

You can adjust the workout, weight, and intensity based on your fitness level and goals.

Listen to your body and take rest days if necessary.

Upcoming Week: As you enter the final week of your challenge, stay motivated and celebrate your progress!

 Keep pushing yourself and enjoy the journey!

CHAPTER 7

YOU DID IT!-_celebrate success and look to the future_

Congratulations!

You've reached the final chapter of the 28 Day Fitness Challenge!

This incredible journey may have transformed your physical health, boosted your confidence and sparked a sense of accomplishment.

Take a moment to acknowledge the hard work, dedication, and positive changes you've made.

Reflect on your journey: Review your goals: What were your initial goals for the challenge?

Have you reached them yet?

How have your goals evolved throughout the program?

Challenges and Triumphs: What are some of the challenges you face and how do you overcome them? Celebrate your wins, big and small!

Favorite aspect: What aspect of the program did you find most beneficial?

Have you discovered any new exercises or activities that you love?

Overall Progress: How has your overall fitness and health improved?

Have you noticed any changes in strength, endurance or energy levels?

Maintain momentum: Overcome challenges The key to lasting results is maintaining healthy habits beyond 28 days.

Here are some tips to stay motivated and on track:

Set SMART goals: Set goals that are specific, measurable, attainable, relevant, and time-bound time to stay focused and motivated.

Find a workout partner: Having a workout partner can provide support, accountability and make exercise more enjoyable.

Schedule your workouts: Treat your workouts like important appointments and schedule them in your calendar.

Consistency is key!

Mix up your routine: Explore new activities or change up your existing routine to avoid boredom and continue to challenge yourself.

Reward yourself: Celebrate milestones and achievements along the way.

A new workout outfit, a massage, or a fun activity can be great motivators.

Listen to your body: Plan your rest days and incorporate recovery strategies like stretching and foam rolling to avoid exhaustion and injury.

Find an activity you love: Fitness doesn't have to be a chore.

Explore different activities until you find what you really enjoy.

Looking Ahead: Your Fitness Journey Continues The 28 Day Challenge has equipped you with the tools and knowledge to live a healthier lifestyle.

Remember, fitness is a lifelong journey, not a destination.

Challenge yourself, explore new activities and most importantly have fun!

This program is just the beginning of an exciting journey towards a healthier, happier life.

INDEX

- Achievements
- Active Recovery
- Challenges
- Consistency
- Flexibility
- Goals
- Habits
- Mindset
- Nutrition
- Progress
- Support
- Sustainability
- Well-being

Dear valued readers, your feedback is invaluable! After my book, please take a moment to leave a review. Your thoughts help me grow as an author. Thank you